Over-coming Clumsiness

PHYSICAL DEXTERITY
FOR PEOPLE
WHO THOUGHT
IT WAS IMPOSSIBLE

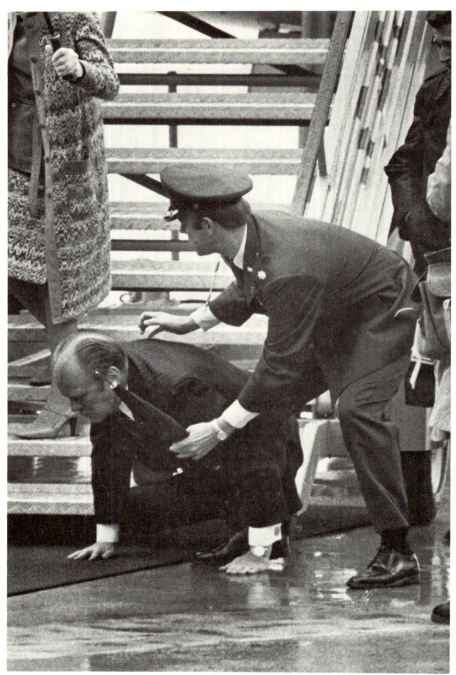

"Even the mightiest have fallen."

OVER-COMING CLUMSINESS

PHYSICAL DEXTERITY FOR PEOPLE WHO THOUGHT IT WAS IMPOSSIBLE

David Lynn Chandler
Jonathan Eisen

Photography by J.B. Grant

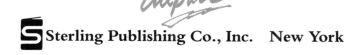

Sterling Publishing Co., Inc.   New York

Library of Congress Cataloging-in-Publication Data

Chandler, David Lynn.
  Overcoming clumsiness.

  "A Sterling impact book."
  Includes index.
  1. Clumsiness—Popular works.   I. Eisen, Jonathan.
II. Title.
RC925.5.C48 1986   152.3'85   85-31730
ISBN 0-8069-6348-4
ISBN 0-8069-6350-6 (pbk.)

Copyright © 1986 by David Lynn Chandler, Jonathan Eisen, and J. B. Grant
Published by Sterling Publishing Co., Inc.
Two Park Avenue, New York, N.Y. 10016
Distributed in Australia by Capricorn Book Co. Pty. Ltd.
Unit 5C1 Lincoln St., Lane Cove, N.S.W. 2066
Distributed in the United Kingdom by Blandford Press
Link House, West Street, Poole, Dorset BH15 1LL, England
Distributed in Canada by Oak Tree Press Ltd.
% Canadian Manda Group, P.O. Box 920, Station U
Toronto, Ontario, Canada M8Z 5P9
Manufactured in the United States of America
All rights reserved

Table of Contents

Frontispiece, 2
Preface, 6
Introduction, 7
Controlling Accidents, 11
Self-Evaluation, 16
Proving, 18
Proving II, 20
Desk Set, 22
Coordinating, 24
Forgiveness, 26
Balance, 27
Balance II, 29
Balance III, 30
Overcompensating, 32
Introspection, 34
Blockage, 35
Labels, 36
Too Busy, 38
Inhibition, 39
All Thumbs, 40
Fear, 43
Slipping, 44
Falling, 46
Hemispheric Dominance, 48

Head Bumping, 52
Fire, 54
The Breath, 56
Breathing, 57
Paralysis, 58
Releasing Anger, 59
Chaos, 61
Murphy's Law, 64
Circulatory Stagnancy, 66
Circulatory Stagnancy II, 69
Losing, 70
Guilt, 72
Embarrassment, 73
Timing, 75
Timing II, 76
Timing III, 78
Not Listening, 81
Habit, 82
Tension in the Arms, 84
Lateness, 88
Going Unconscious, 88
Masks, 90
About the Authors, 95
Index, 96

Preface

"If you accept your limitations you get to keep them."—Robbie Gass

This is a book about overcoming clumsiness. It is also about overcoming self-limitations. Clumsiness arises out of your thoughts as much as it does from your body. If you can alter your thoughts—especially those you have about yourself—you can alter your clumsiness and transform it into gracefulness and agility. Although this is a book of exercises, it is also a book about *personal* transformation. It is a book about how to move without fear; it is a book about change.

Words like *clumsy* and *graceful* reflect not only a physicality but also an orientation that comes from an autobiographical pattern of interaction with the world. Many of the exercises and affirmations in this book are about breaking negative patterns and replacing them with more useful ones. Regardless of how much you may agree or disagree with what is written here, nothing can be accomplished unless you actually move from opinion to action.

By reading this book you are making a beginning in a process of change. Do not look for a quick fix, a miracle cure, or instantaneous transformation. Whatever happens will be the direct result of your dedication. We can only serve you as guides. Remember to be gentle and patient and above all, loving. Everything in this book has been tested, and proven. All it needs now to be complete is you.

There is no special order for the exercises, but we suggest that whatever you start with, start slowly. Do what you can and each time try to do more. Never strain. Always relax. Chart your improvement; enjoy it all.

David Chandler
Jonathan Eisen

Brotherhood of the Inept

By David Binder

Probably it runs in the family, this clumsiness, not as a river but at least as a stream enveloping one of us each generation. My father held on to a garage door handle after he had pulled it down. It slammed on his thumb. He fell off a bicycle and broke his arm. Once, when my mother threw a dress-up luncheon party in our backyard for his business colleagues, a tablecloth concealed a large irregularity on the edge of our rustic table. It was at this spot that my father, wearing a white suit, placed his plate of spaghetti with tomato sauce. It toppled into his lap. He changed into another white suit, sat down at the same place and spilled a second plate. Changing again upstairs, he dropped his pocket watch on the tile floor of the bathroom. It stopped.

One wet and icy February, the roof above our living room began to leak. In a business suit, my father mounted a ladder carrying a claw hammer. Losing his footing, he desperately pounded the claw through the asphalt shingles the way an Alpine climber uses an ice ax. He broke through the ceiling, and the leak increased.

These incidents amused the members of our family and gave me a brief and dangerous sense of superiority. Had I not recognized, at the relatively late age of 12, that I was heir to the clumsy streak? Had the significance of my inability to throw a basketball through a hoop, much less dribble it, escaped me?

One day a friend took me along to a country club to work for him as a caddy. Golf was more alien to me than Albania. My first and last golfer asked for "a wood." I handed him a 5-iron. We reached the first green and he prepared to putt. I held the flag stick firmly in the hole. The ball hit the pole and bounced off. He cursed: "Clumsy!" I have kept my distance from the game these 43 years.

At this distance, I can observe that what distinguishes the clumsy from the graceful is our total inability to recognize the functions at which we will surely fail—dancing, fancy diving, sanding wood, catching a fly ball or carrying a glass safely to a table. In high school, where sports were compulsory, I volunteered to dive for the swimming team, knowing, at least, that I would be a poor racer. I could never sufficiently coordinate two arm movements with two leg movements. I can still hear the voice through the loudspeaker announcing: "Binder will attempt a one-and-a-half gainer with a half twist." I lifted off the board, went into wild contortions and landed on my back, splashing the onlookers. I stayed for a time at the bottom of the pool, but when I finally surfaced they were still laughing. I retreated to the cross-country team.

In retrospect, it is the not-knowing that is so galling to the clumsy: not knowing when and where we are going to lumber. A modest facility at playing the clarinet or typing or even getting down a hill on skis is liable to seduce us into feeling that we may have overcome terminal awkwardness. Down this path, and not very far down it, lies a branch over which we will trip.

After years of summers paddling canoes and portaging them on narrow trails, I fancied myself handy with this mode of transportation. Not so. With my father in a canoe, I tipped over on a placid stretch of the upper Wisconsin River, prompting him, of all persons, to brand me: "Clumsy!" Recently I capsized a canoe while trying to retrieve a fishing lure that was snagged on a tree limb, dumping an old friend into the drink. Soon after, my friend lost his glasses. He, too, may belong to the brotherhood of the inept, but it is a mark of the clumsy not to be able to discern the trait readily in others.

When two clumsy persons get together, cataclysm is not far away. Once I was teasing my father in the presence of two of my friends. He playfully threw a short, clumsy punch that caught me in the stomach, sending me reeling across the room and slumping to the floor. My father and I were quite surprised at this sudden confluence of our mutual in-coordination. My friends thought it was hilarious.

There is a blitheness that attends being clumsy. My father, for instance, floored the brake pedal of the family car at a crossroad where there was a conspicuous amount of loose gravel on the asphalt. The car spun completely around and ended up facing in the direction my father wished to go. His passenger, on leave after being wounded in the Africa campaign of World War II, was frightened more, he said, than by anything he had experienced in the desert fighting. Father only smiled and remarked: "Didn't I do that nicely?"

With the passage of much time, a degree of awareness may accumulate for the clumsy. Thus, I watched with a kind of eerie contentment as a recent house guest walked straight into our glass porch door twice within 10 minutes. I was also able to appreciate the story of Vasil Bilak, the Czechoslovak Communist Politburo member whose proof of proletarian genuineness was displayed a few years ago at an exhibition commemorating the 60th anniversary of the founding of his ruling party in Prague. It was his certificate as a journeyman tailor from a town in Moravia, dated 1926. For 10 crowns, a museum guard slipped the parchment out of its frame and displayed the reverse side. On it, the master tailor who examined young Bilak had written: "He is all right on the trousers, but don't let him at the jackets."

But awareness has its limits. So I go on determinedly felling trees on power lines, painting windows shut, bumping people on dance floors, sawing crookedly and spilling sugar. Those, at least, are the clumsinesses I remember, but there may be thousands I never even noticed. My wife is plainly sympathetic, maybe even empathetic. After I sharpen the kitchen knives, invariably nicking them, she usually cuts herself.

Perhaps recognition of clumsiness is at the root of my occasional dream of having only to take a deep breath to be able to rise unaided toward the heavens and, with a few deft hand movements, to fly to an altitude of about 500 feet. No one else is up there with me, and those graceful tennis players, golfers and fly fishermen I can still see below are in awe of my gracefulness. In that dream I am never clumsy.

David Binder *is assistant news editor in the Washington bureau of The New York Times.* (Reprinted by permission.)

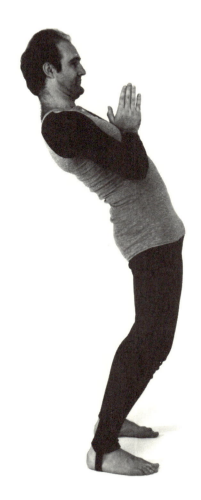

Palms together at chest height, bend backwards. Hold it. Straighten up. Do it again. It's not as easy as you think.

Controlling Accidents

This year millions of people will injure themselves in so-called accidents. Are you one of them? Will you cut yourself, fall, drop things, bump into other people, drive into another car? Regardless of what you call these events, only a small percentage of them will be caused by mechanical failures or the vicissitudes of nature—circumstances over which you as an individual have absolutely no control. You can control "accidents."

Leaving out industrial accidents, where genuinely hazardous conditions predominate, a large number of accidents are preventable. They are events over which you have some measure of control, and "somehow" you do not exercise it. Are you one of those who for a variety of reasons disclaim responsibility—and attribute your clumsiness to "inevitability?" Do you dislike acknowledging that your very thoughts may be responsible for creating some of the conditions that "befall" you?

Even the nomenclature of accidents may bespeak a certain passivity, as in the very term "accident," which *happens to* people who are "accident-prone" or who have "bad luck." Why do "accidents" happen to you?

Some people just can't get into a car without bumping their heads or sit down at a table without spilling soup on themselves. Still others are the elderly who resign themselves as time goes by to less and less agility, coordination or strength. For them, infirmity is something that just "naturally" happens as a result of getting older. Advancing years are thought of as a path to lessening ability, greater stiffness and fragility—regardless of the example of legions of older people who are living examples of health and vigor and who do not necessarily decline as the years go by.

The problem, it seems, is not in the stars—to paraphrase Shakespeare—but in ourselves, in our thinking. We do not take responsibility for our thoughts, as though someone else were thinking them, someone else creating our reality for us.

This does not mean that suddenly "believing" that you are strong or agile will make it so. If you have allowed your body to calcify and stiffen, positive thinking won't make it supple and strong.

What we mean is that in time your thoughts tend to create "reality" and that your predisposition to reality can determine—to a large extent—your future. If you believe that old age is a time of infirmity and accidents, broken hips and declining health, this can predetermine what you do with your body on the way to old age. All prophecy is to a degree self-fulfilling, and most of us "prove" our beliefs about old age when we get there.

On the other side, believing that life is to be lived and enjoyed to the fullest in good health can create the conditions under which that really happens, well into old age.

For people who are clumsy, the same holds true. Clumsiness may be manifested by the body but it often starts in the mind. An understanding of some of the roots of clumsiness can help you achieve a dexterity long thought to be an impossible dream . . . that is, provided you begin to develop a more positive relationship with your body.

The purpose of this book is to give you an opportunity to overcome your own personal "Klutz." Included are numerous exercises that if followed diligently and patiently will allow you to have a safe relationship with other humans, with animals and inanimate objects. But before we even begin to discuss any exercises, a few more words are in order on the importance and role of attitudes.

Clumsiness is an attitude problem as much as it is a physical "disability." Attitudes—or thoughts—about your body and its relationship to the world largely determine who you become and how you get there. Webster defines *klutz* not only as a clumsy person but also a "wooden block." How does a baby born with such amazing flexibility and strength mutate into a wooden block over time, blundering into danger, "unconsciously" producing pain and injury?

For many, the world first presents itself as a life-threatening menace. Coming from the perfection of the womb, many people are birthed quite painfully by insensitive obstetricians. First breaths are drawn in response to a painful slap. Or sometimes, the umbilical cord is cut before breathing begins, throwing the infant into panic. The first message here is, "I am going to die." Also: "Breathing equals pain," and "The world is threatening." We begin to "hold on" for dear life, often holding on to our breath for security.

As babies grow into their two's and three's, the world amplifies its danger again, just at the point when babies begin experimenting with newly-sensed dexterity and independence. Restrictions are imposed in the face of the very young, and physical experimentation is often countered by parents eager to preserve the child's physical safety and/or infancy. Early touching/manipulation forays are quickly forbidden, and although this urge dies hard, it does die, and along with it often dies the enthusiasm of early curiosity. Physical retardation is often the result, as the child soon learns it gets rewarded for being "well-behaved" and censured for being a searcher/experimenter.

The adult world, hassled as it is, seems to spend decreasing amounts of time nurturing the young. Early authority lessons are frequently accompanied by rage and fury from harassed, frustrated grown-ups, who direct their frustrations at their little children. At this point, many children actually begin to hold their breath in terror and "leave" their body. A feeling of danger burrows in as a "free floating" anxiety, and the child's body coils back into a fetal position during sleep. Over time, the breathing gets shallower, partly held during stressful and non-stressful situations alike. The young person begins living everywhere but in the present—in past traumas, future dreams, wishes and fantasies. The body is left to fend for itself, and breathing, which can process anxiety (witness the function of the sigh), becomes paralyzed. The whole person becomes paralyzed in a sense as well, freezing anxiety patterns throughout the body; these become manifest in tension and numerous allied diseases.

The child begins to take on the characteristics of the clumsy—largely because he/she is living in two different places at the same time—a fantasy place that is safe (removed from the trauma-inducing "real world") and the physical place whose attributes are often ignored.

After situations of profoundly negative intensity, children sometimes never entirely return to their body. They go unconscious in various realms of their own existence, yielding control to whatever happens. They literally become "out of touch" with their own lives. The patterns of clumsiness are rooted here. The physical world becomes not a learning forum but as something from which to escape. Mistakes are not accepted as part of learning experience, but as something for which to be punished, and all too often the flickering light of curiosity goes out forever.

One more essential aspect of the attitudinal realm of clumsiness is related to the deprivation of love that many children encounter. This can profoundly affect the development of physical agility.

When a child experiences a scarcity of love from parents, he/she develops a concept that the whole world lacks enough love—and from there he/she begins to try to elicit the missing love through a number of strategies. Many people begin a life of clumsiness by trying to obtain the love they need through injury or illness (real or faked). For many, the sickbed is one of the few genuinely nurturing places of childhood. An injury evokes genuine expressions of concern/love, and many resort to this device as an "unconscious" love-seeking strategy. This continues on through marriage and later life. Some children crave attention so badly that they injure themselves often enough to develop a life-long pattern. Sometimes, unconscious self-inflicted injury merely reflects a negative self-estimation. This may be brought about by love deprivation, and it usually appears to be associated with love-attraction strategies, the plan being to recapture the nurturing they received as children, using their spouse (or whoever else is handy) as a substitute parent.

For every Klutz who injures or disables himself in order to elicit love, there is the Klutz who tries to please everyone *else* in order to elicit love. Such a person seems to exist for everyone other than him/herself. This person does not really act from a generosity of spirit but rather from a conditioned pattern derived from trying to please an unpleasable parent/elder. This parent/elder usually required "respect" but would not be satisfied *no matter what the child did*. This is part of the "not-enough" syndrome—something that results from finding that nothing could please the adult, that is, short of the child's hurting or stunting him/herself.

People who grow up in this kind of situation frequently produce accidents in their need for validation for their "givingness." Personal laws such as "I hurt myself trying to give to others" tend to heighten their sense of martyrdom, thereby "proving" what good people they really are. Since the parent never recognized or rewarded them enough, or loved them enough, in later life the reward is sought in the sympathy and gratitude from people not fully aware of the motivation for the "giving." Such a person wants to be loved and appreciated through service, and failing to achieve that will get it any way possible, often through self-inflicted pain.

What about the elderly? For many older people bad health, fragility and declining dexterity are seen as "natural." The harder it is to get out of bed, the more time they spend there. In a downwards spiral, physical decline and decreasing motivation feed one another, each one seen as "normal." For younger generations, old age is also seen as a time of declining health and vitality, despite the evidence of millions of older people who live out their years in good health and vitality. In this mind-set, these people are seen as "exceptions" rather than as examples of the fact that your life is what you make of it and that old age, like any age, can be patterned after your highest expectations. Again, it is the thought that counts.

To what extent can you actually take responsibility for your thoughts? Most people have a hard time merely taking responsibility for their actions. When confronted with evidence of their "unconscious" motivations for self-inflicted injury—accidents over which they do have some control—they might find themselves reliving some past negativity. Moreover, they may find here the beginnings of elaborate compensatory mechanisms, evasions or disassociations from their early painful memories.

Taking responsibility for your thoughts means replacing trauma-induced patterns founded in the "not-enough" syndrome with thoughts based on a more realistic assessment of the Universe-as-it-is. This begins with the acknowledgment that you have more to do with your injuries—and their avoidance—than you might have previously admitted. Patterns of negativity can be reversed, but the belief that they are indelible helps you to keep them. We hope that the progress that can be demonstrated by using the information in this book will help alter this belief, beginning the process of unravelling some of the more persistent negative belief/behavior patterns.

Overcoming accidents and physical clumsiness begins with the recognition of the power we all have, whether or not we are aware of it, *whether or not we have ever used it in a conscious way.* It means returning to the body with love, and letting go of fear is a good first step. Taking responsibility for one's thoughts can be very frightening at first, but only because of the realization of how much power we actually have over our own lives.

Self-Evaluation

This book will help you build a more empowered state of being. In order to become happier and experience less suffering you must necessarily evaluate your entire life including the past, the present, and the future.

The past has brought you to where you are now in the present. The present takes you to where you will be in the future. The essence of change takes place in the *now*. This is the only moment that can effectively change your life. Putting off to tomorrow is the refuge of sin and procrastination and therefore keeps you stuck in past mistakes and repetition of blunders and pain.

Evaluating what you are doing now and what you have done in the past to bring you to this very moment in your life enables you to examine the pattern of your own thinking. Observation, as any good scientist will tell you, creates a change in the observed. So by examining your past and witnessing your past choices you can begin to evolve into a new awareness, strengthening your talents towards change.

Exercises

1. Sitting comfortably in a chair or on the floor, with your spine erect, close your eyes and recall all the events in your life when you have been in some accident or some difficulty. Bring the memories back as precisely as you can. See what is around you in the environment. Feel the texture of the objects around you. Smell the odors in the area. Taste the taste you sense in your mouth. Listen to the sounds you hear in the environment. Now get in touch with what it was that saved you from being in worse condition than you actually were in. What protected you?

2. Repeat this exercise, but this time recall all your moments of great physical ability. Recreate the feeling of being bright and powerful and graceful. Bring back the physical memory of sensations that gave you these feelings of happiness and confidence.

3. Now go back to the "bad times" and *change them*. Using your imagination, pretend that what you did "wrong" you are now able to change by making a different choice. See, feel, hear, taste, smell the difference in the situation as you now have corrected it. How do you feel? People unconsciously alter the past in their memories of pain all the time. The reason we are doing this now is that we are doing it *consciously*. To paraphase George Orwell, he who can control the past controls the future.

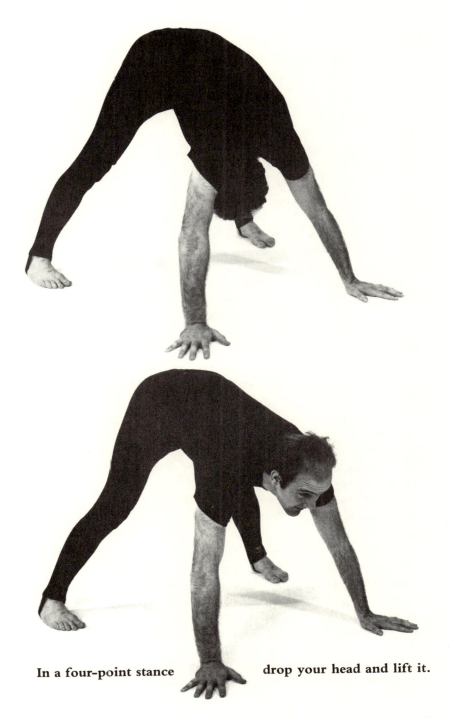

In a four-point stance   drop your head and lift it.

Proving

Being able to "take" physical punishment is in many cultures seen as the measure of masculinity. Injuries are seen as badges of one's manhood, and in the teen years especially, there is a certain satisfaction in being carried off the field after a play. After a time, a positive association grows between injury and psychic reward, enhanced by the admiration of your fellow males, as well as the motherly ministrations of adoring females.

Eventually, possibly even in early childhood, the male becomes "enarmored" with himself, hardening his psychic repertoire, ruling out "softness" as unmasculine. *The seven-year-old turned from his mother's kisses, looked helplessly skyward. "Please, Mom," he said, turning away from her, embarrassed.*

Although many toughened males become supremely well coordinated, many do not. Many never make the full connection to their softer half, their *anima*, and never attain the grace that comes from living completely. The cloture that occurs in early childhood creates a lasting impression on the adult psyche, closing men off to their bodies—except in acts of conquest, which often includes sex. Cut off from their bodies, some men fail to receive pleasure through their bodies which eventually drop away from them for lack of love or attention.

Men generally think they have to prove themselves in a dog-eat-dog world and, rather than work together to end human suffering, they compete for personal gain at the expense of others. It is still the Middle Ages, and excuses abound.

The Klutz is somewhat like a soccer player who refuses to pass off to a teammate, losing the goal because he is headstrong and unwilling to give ground in order to attain the goal. Throughout the ages, the bending reed has been a symbol of strength through flexibility, as opposed to the unbending rod that breaks in the wind. Refusing to yield when yielding is appropriate not only increases frustration: it increases the rage inside. The desire to prove yourself increases and becomes more difficult to control.

Achieving the fullness of life goes beyond mere survival to the realm of complete aliveness and the expression of one's freedom.

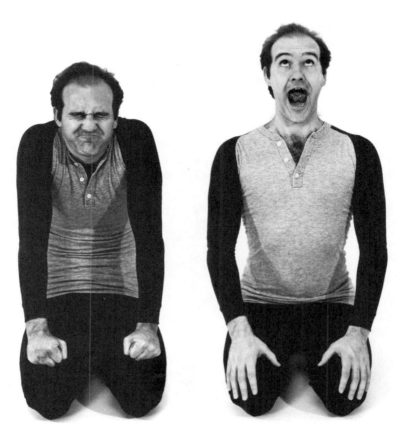

Open your mouth and eyes to the most extreme, then close them to the most extreme. This relaxes the face and releases "proving" poses.

Affirmation
I have nothing to prove. The Universe loves me as I am.

Exercise
The really macho men confront their fears head on. If you are afraid to appear emotional, vulnerable and loving, confront the fear and how you react to it.

Proving II

This exercise is helpful for releasing the need to prove one's sex. This helps rid the male of having to prove that he is macho and tough and powerful, and vice versa for the female. Pretend you are the opposite sex and be the archetypal opposite. Really do it up. Play as if you are the sexiest opposite that you can imagine.

Now pretend you are the most powerful same sex and feel the difference. What is the difference to you? Ask yourself what it is you have to prove and to whom you have to prove it, and let it go. Affirm that you do not have to prove anything to anyone. "I am perfect the way I am and any changes I make are choices of increase."

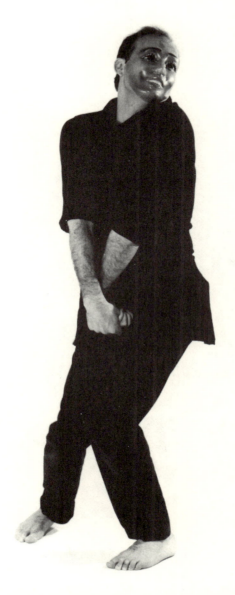

Masks are good tools for overcoming embarrassment. Try playing the person the mask depicts.

Desk Set

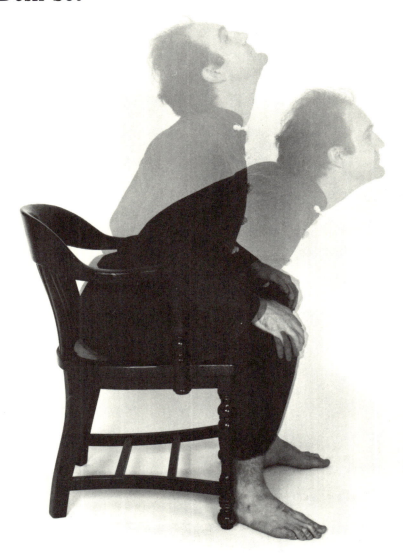

While sitting at a desk, rock forward and back with your face and head looking to the ceiling as you lean forward and looking to the ground as you curve back and lean in the other direction. This "s" shape that changes to a "c" shape can help enliven the spine and wake up the system and rid the body and mind of tension.

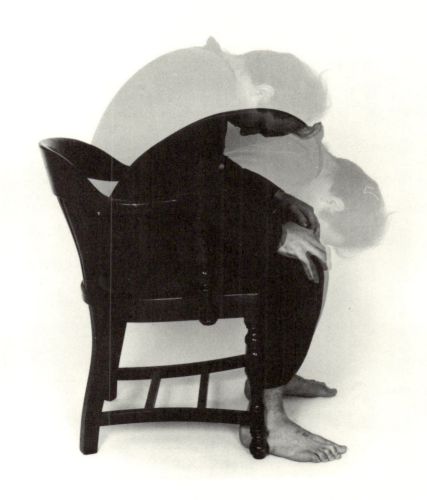

Coordinating

Sitting, gently pound your leg with your fist in an up-and-down motion. With your other hand rub your other thigh. Then switch hands. Switch back and forth and keep the actions separate. One hand is a fist up and down in a soft hitting fashion while the other is a rubbing motion sliding along the thigh. Keep switching faster and faster.

Hold a bucket full of water. Change hands. Pour it very slowly into the tub or sink. Watch how the water moves and how it flows and seeks the lowest place to move to and collects itself when it has nowhere else to flow.

Imitate the movement of the water. Use your arms and your legs and your whole body. Take two glasses, one full of water and the other empty and pour the full into the empty. Continue this back-and-forth movement of the fluid and imagine that you are the fluid. Keep as much of the fluid from spilling as you can. Imitate this movement.

Take a handful of earth and knead it with your hands. Play with it and smell it. Watch how it reacts to your touch. When you imitate the earth, feel the weight of it and its heaviness and its strength. Let that "groundness" be part of you.

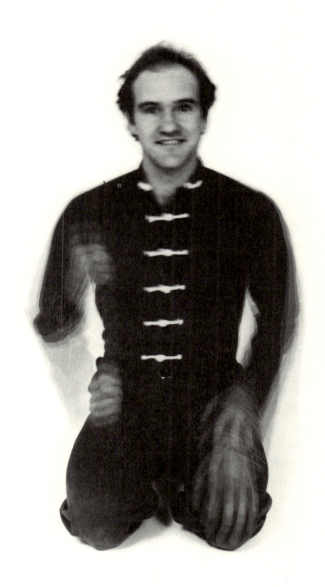

Forgiveness

To err is human, to forgive, divine. These words are the cornerstone to the transformation that is possible. When the Klutz forgives himself and others he can become graceful, open and liquid in movement, because he has become graceful in his heart and mind. What is forgiveness? *To give as before*—to give as before something happened that made you *not* want to give any more. How do you forgive? Forgiveness is a cessation of resentment, a giving up of claims against an offender. You forgive by practicing giving, by practicing letting go.

Exercises

1. Give a present to the person you want to forgive.
2. Give yourself a present.
3. Say to the offender "I forgive you for . . . ."
4. Say to yourself "I forgive you for . . . ."
5. Throw a party for all the people you have not forgiven and make little treats for all of them concerning the offenses they committed.
6. Play with your offenders. Push them and pull them around the space. Let them know what you are doing and why.
7. Let your feelings of love return and express them to your friend.
8. Consider what would have happened if you were on the other side of the offense. Put yourself in the offender's shoes.
9. Standing on your bed or near it, give in to gravity and fall on the bed.
10. Tell the story of the event as if you were the other person. and ask for forgiveness.
11. Standing with the person you want to forgive play give and take by alternately pushing and pulling each other in a semi-embrace.
12. Declare your forgiveness of yourself to another. Let others declare their forgiveness of themselves. Encourage your friends.

Balance I

When you free your physical body you free your mind. When you elevate the physical experience of your body you elevate the mental experience of the mind. Freedom, is both physical and mental. When we are able to alter one we alter the other automatically. Clumsiness comes from mental and physical imbalance. Imbalance comes from a feeling of unsteadiness and "ungroundedness." When you increase balance and groundedness you have the sensation of freedom and express yourself in grace and ease. The results of balance are joy and friendliness.

Exercises

1. Stand on one leg for as long as you can. Switch legs.

2. Rock back on your heels. Rock forward onto your toes. Do this with increasing motion until your body almost goes off-balance.

3. Rock from side to side with increasing magnitude, getting just to the brink of going off balance, but never beyond it.

4. Pretend you are on a tightrope. Walk across the room on a straight line. Pretend that there's no net, and that you have to get to the other side as fast as possible. If you fall off, you have to start over.

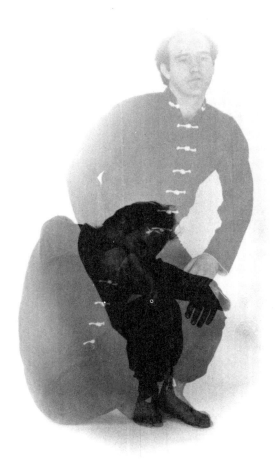

From a seated position (cross-legged) stand up without using the hands. This promotes strength and balance in the legs, back and stomach.

Balance II

Problems of clumsiness are often associated with a lack of balance, itself often the result of a lack of "connection" with the middle ear. Frequently this lack of balance is associated with high or low blood pressure, middle ear dysfunctions, concussions or tumors. Sometimes nutritional deficiencies are implicated; sometimes the problem is neurological; sometimes alcohol is at the root. If you suspect that your balance problems are associated with any of these causes, or are caused by bifocals, you should consult a physician.

If your problems persist after clearing your medical check-up, you may be wise to try some of the following exercises which are designed to help you establish a better working relationship with your body.

Exercises

1. Stand on one foot, then the other. While standing, raise one leg at a time to your chest, holding the knees with both hands.

2. Lying on your stomach on your floor or bed, bend your legs up from the knees. Then start crossing them, back and forth. This activates the muscles and nerves in the lower back.

3. Ballroom dancing can be fun and help coordination.

4. Foot massage is an excellent way to get to a more friendly relationship with your feet. Feel for places of tension and pain. Massage them away with the thumb, knuckles or even a wooden foot roller, something that can be kept under your desk and used throughout the day.

5. Balance a book on your head and walk around the room!

Balance III

Another exercise from which one can acquire balance is to actually do some spinning. This is best done with a partner to help keep you safe from falling during your first few times out with this exercise. Make sure you have plenty of room to move around and there are no sharp corners near you.

Look at the palm of your hand and never look away from it during the entire course of this exercise. In spinning, this is very important for if you look away you may become extremely dizzy and you might even fall down. As a child you might have played at spinning in circles until you fell down but you must not give in to the temptation to get dizzy or fall down.

Continuing to look at the palm of the right hand, spin in the direction of your thumb. With your right hand palm up towards your face you should spin to the right. Go very slowly at first and take your time building up your speed. You will find that you will want to go faster and faster, but control this urge so that you won't lose your balance by getting dizzy. If you get dizzy, don't stop! Keep looking at your HAND and slowly slow down. Once you have gone from a standstill to a point of speed that feels exhilarating, then you can experiment with spinning in the other direction. Experiment with switching directions, looking at the other hand immediately and going the other way. The switching procedure increases your ability to adapt to the change of your inner ear fluid and lets you keep more control over yourself, giving you a brand-new sense of yourself.

Many people feel like they are re-experiencing their childhood; others feel that they have suddenly discovered the center of their being. Still others find that they are surprised that they can communicate with the outside world more readily as a result of spinning. A note on the hand that is trailing: Just let it hang and it will find its own place in the movement. Primarily that place will be hanging slightly down, so that one hand will be pointing predominantly up and the other hanging mostly towards the ground.

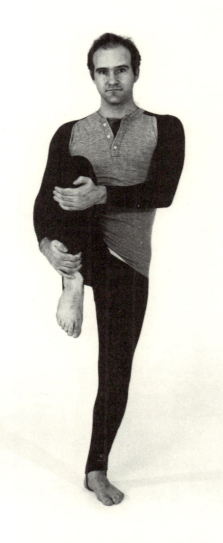

Standing on one foot, bring knee to chest. This promotes balance, gives the lower back a good stretch, gets you up and moving. This can be done in your office without attracting undue attention.

Overcompensating

The Klutz rarely takes the time to do the little things right, rushing on to the next thing before insuring that the last thing was accomplished. The goal is more conscious control—more awareness about what you are doing and how you are doing it. Accidents are the result of going unconscious, losing that awareness. Do you walk around life with a great deal of "noise" in your head? Are you less than 100 percent in the moment? Do you allow your "unconscious" to rule your waking moments and are you continually surprised by what you have done?

The unconscious can be thought of as everything that is not conscious, rather than as some dark, unfathomable place, dank and mysterious. Some of the exercises in this book will give you a greater access to the unconscious as repression of uncomfortable memories no longer seems desirable. Living in the world is not so terrible. Besides, consider the alternative!

If you let your repressed, or unconscious, desires and/or fears rule your daily life, you often overcompensate for felt needs, or desires. A more fully awake, alive, conscious person will have less need for repression, more ability to be 100 percent in the moment. You will have less need to go overboard to express strength because there will be less felt/perceived weakness.

Overcompensating takes place when you feel inferior or guilty or inadequate. It comes as an excessive reaction to a stimulus. When you overcompensate you are *indulging in clumsiness*. We all feel inadequate at times. This is exactly the time to be wary of the Klutz preparing to strike. It is often hard to recognize when you begin to go overboard in your reactions to events but there are many telltale signs. When you recognize these signs you can begin to find your balance in the situation and avoid clumsiness.

Exercises

1. When in a conversation with a friend check to see if the communication is balanced. Are you talking too much? Are you interrupting? Are you talking too fast? Balance the situation by checking your rate of speed and the length of each statement in your conversation.

2. Set a small goal in relation to any person with whom you feel a sense of inadequacy. For instance, move a little closer to the person. Make the movement very small. Continue to move toward them in very minute movements. Notice if your movements are too abrupt. Slowly you will begin to see that you can actually move the other person across the room at a very small rate of speed. In doing this you will gain a greater amount of physical control. You will prove to yourself that you are able to be effective with this person.

3. Repeat the small moves but now move slightly backwards instead of forwards. How does this make you feel?

4. Slow down and take a deep breath whenever you are with the people who bring up your feelings of guilt of inadequacy.

5. Affirm to yourself that you are indeed adequate to deal with the situation.

6. Comparing yourself to others brings you into contention with them. If you feel they are "better," you will feel small. If you feel they are "worse," you will feel arrogant. Choose to see others as equal to yourself. Visualize when you are in conversation that you are looking at yourself and that you are equal to yourself. How does this make you feel?

Introspection

What would happen if your every deed were recorded somewhere and that at the end of your life you could look back at this recording and view every little action you had ever taken? Think about that for a moment. If every little movement and every little sound, taste, touch, feeling, everything, were recorded, would you be likely to change the things you do now? Well, guess what? They *are* all recorded inside you. Somewhere inside, you have recorded in memory and kinesthetic awareness everything you have ever done and everything you have ever known. If you look at yourself in this way you can begin to see that you actually do have many choices in life and also see where you have created your own clumsiness. The one overriding purpose for clumsiness is to learn. Mistakes are for learning. If you do not learn from your mistakes you will continue to make them.

Exercises

1. Pay attention to every move you make for the next half hour. Pretend you are making a mental note of everything you do. Watch yourself and listen to everything you do. Can you hear your breathing? Can you feel the ground beneath your feet? Do you go away from yourself, and forget the exercise? What are your thoughts? What has changed from the time you started watching?

2. Now shift your focus from observing yourself to observing another person. Record everything that they are doing. Ask yourself what they are feeling. Ask what they are paying attention to. If they notice your observation, what changes in them? Can you hear their breathing? Do they appear to sense the ground under their feet? What is happening to you as you are observing them? All of this gives you "extra" consciousness.

Blockage

Clumsiness is blockage. Overcoming any blockage will decrease whatever clumsiness you may experience.

Exercises

1. To unblock your stomach area and liver and create a greater flow, rub your belly area in a circular fashion in a clockwise direction. Start on the outer edges of the belly and move in smaller circles into the middle. Start in the middle and move in a counterclockwise direction, letting the circles increase in size as you go outwards.

2. Kidneys overworked by too much coffee or drinking can be helped by massaging them with the fists. Rub the back just under the ribs in a circular movement. This also revitalizes the adrenal glands.

3. In the middle of the chest, use the knuckle on your thumb to rub in very small circles. This invigorates the thymus gland.

4. Using the thumbs of both hands, massage the occipital buns (the little muscles that sit at the base of the skull). This can sometimes alleviate headaches, and release the tensions that may come from working for too long in a sitting position.

Labels

Once you accept the Klutz label, it often becomes a self-fulfilling prophecy. A fellow of about twelve, going through that awkward stage of development that bridges the gap between the child and the adolescent, received the nickname "Crash" because he was accident-prone. Since he was expected to fumble about, he frequently did. Most of the time this came from the expectation that he internalized of his own predisposition towards clumsiness. The truth of the matter was that he was simply nervous and this fed his awkwardness. He had accepted the notion that he was a Klutz and he continually "proved" it.

This kind of labelling occurs more often than you might suspect, perhaps even in your case, and it can affect your self-image profoundly.

The label that you have come to accept may become more you than you. In order to overcome this, take the time to examine the labels that you have accepted from others and the ones you now own. Are you comfortable with these labels? Do they enhance your self-image? Do they conflict with your sense of who you would like to be? Do the labels help you or do they keep you confined? If they are confining and debilitating, rid yourself of them. Refuse to accept the label, see it as an insult to your higher self that you wish to express and confront the persons who are attaching these labels to you. Accepting a label means you get to keep it. When you allow people to put you in a limited state of mind you are allowing them to control you, and limit you.

Exercises

1. Write down all the names that you are called. Write down all the labels that you have accepted in your life. Write down all the labels that you have not accepted but that continue to stick to you.

2. Write down all the opposites to the above lists. Everything that you have been labelled has an opposite and that is what you also are. If you have been labelled a goody-goody all your life there must also be some part of you that is perhaps a baddy-baddy. Explore the possibilities of these opposites of your accepted labels.

3. Write down all the labels that you would like to have attached to you. Now write down all the opposites to these.

4. Can you now choose the labels that you absolutely refuse to accept from other people? After you choose these, then you can stop people from making these a part of you by saying, "Please do not call me that again," or "It makes me feel bad when you say that to me," or "What makes you want to categorize me and limit me in that way?" You can choose to empower yourself in a graceful way and express yourself by asking questions and confronting your labellers, telling them about your feelings, about the unconscious labelling that is having a physical result on your movements.

Too Busy

Quiet the mind and open the heart. One of the simplest methods of gaining greater body control and flow is to sit quietly and pay attention to the quiet around you, expressing love to yourself by taking a break. This is easy, but rarely do we actually take real time to sit and do nothing. How do you do nothing? Is nothing something you can "do?" Try it and see for yourself.

Exercises

1. Sit in a comfortable position with your back erect so that your breathing is not constricted. Loosen your belt and collar. Focus your eyes on the ground three feet from you. Breathe easily and naturally. Count your breathing as you inhale. Whenever a thought enters your mind *let it go*. See it, then release it. Whenever you have a thought go back to the first count. Count to ten. Remember that the counting to ten must be done with a cleared mind. Any time a thought comes in, you must stop your count and begin at one again.

2. Sit in a comfortable erect position. Follow the breath with your mind, watching your own thoughts. See the breath as a cycle and a circle.

3. Sit quietly erect. Imagine that you have a light that shines out from your forehead and that without moving your head you can direct this beam to all parts of your body. Every part of your body it touches is filled with light and soon your entire body is full of light.

4. Sitting quietly, imagine that you are the most compassionate being you can think of and let that being look at your body. Let that being speak lovingly from the heart to you. Have a dialogue with this being. Ask the being how you can become healthier and happier and more graceful.

5. Sitting erect, hum to yourself on one note for ten minutes or as long as you like. Let your mind be quiet and your heart open to whatever comes up.

6. Sitting, focus your mind and heart on a loved one and send him or her love like a radio beam from your whole body. Let this beam grow in power and send it to several loved ones. Allow the beam to grow again, and let it cover the entire planet and come back into you. Note what your response is to this and to how your body feels and reacts for the ten minutes after this exercise.

Inhibition

The image you have of yourself is often formed as a result of your family's collective judgments and desires. Conditional love produces people who are less spontaneous than people who received unconditional love as children. Spontaneity is that quality of being in the moment, following inspiration without premeditation, allowing your creative flow to happen without prior restraint. Being spontaneous is being free and self-generating. To increase your freedom to be all these things requires you to improve your self-estimation.

Affirmation

"The whole Universe loves me for exactly who I am. I no longer need validation from my parents, friends or anyone else."

Exercises

1. Following the exercises in the book will increase your sense of freedom. Indeed, if you have gotten this far you will have already set the forces moving towards increasing the pace and quality of your own personal growth.

2. Set this book down and do one thing that has been difficult for you in the past because of feelings of shame or inadequacy. Remember never to hurt yourself or others in the process of self-liberation. Pleasure yourself by giving pleasure to others and watch your feelings of inhibition melt away.

3. Look at yourself naked in a full-length mirror. What can you improve on? Read Ken Dychtwald's book *Bodymind*. What are your feelings of shame and inadequacy?

4. Make funny faces at yourself in a mirror. Note childish feelings being aroused. How did your inhibitions begin? Forgive yourself totally.

All Thumbs

The development of the opposable thumb was on balance an excellent idea, as was fire and the wheel, both of which came later. However, when all the fingers act as thumbs, a person can often drop things that, on hitting the ground, break.

Unless your fingers are used, they get rusty. Problem: How to use your fingers and strengthen them at the same time, when they are not involved in work.

Exercises

1. Hand-to-hand massage. One hand massages the other, pressing, kneading, squeezing, rubbing, interlocking the fingers—anything that brings energy to the hands, increasing circulation and sensitivity. Give the nails a squeeze between the thumb and index finger, too!

2. Squeeze a small rubber ball or tennis ball, all day long, or until bored. Keep the ball in your pocket and squeeze whenever you can.

3. Rubber bands can be looped around different fingers, providing lateral resistance. Move the fingers with the bands on.

4. Learn a musical instrument. Any one will do. Play at any level.

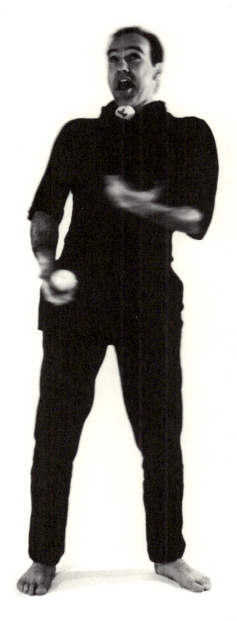

Juggling with one or two or three balls is fun, while promoting physical dexterity, concentration and coordination.

5. Drawing is an excellent way to overcome the problem of all thumbs. By simply sitting in front of a mirror and drawing your own face, you can open yourself to your own self-image, and gradually improve it as you improve your skill. You may not think you can draw, but anyone who can lift a pen or pencil can do this exercise. It does not matter how much experience you have had drawing. Looking in the mirror, trace the outline of your face—without taking your eye from the mirror. This keeps you from judging the accuracy of your effort and maintains your concentration on eye-hand coordination. At the same time you develop an objectivity about your own face.

When you have finished the outline of your face and head, do the hair, eyes, nose and all the features. Remember: *Do not look at the paper and do not take your eyes from the image in the mirror.* Keep your eyes and hand as closely as possibly in synch. When your eyes move, your hand moves. When you have finished your whole face, you may look at the drawing. Do not expect to see a Rembrandt. In fact, the picture may not look like you at all. It may not even look like a person, but that is not the point.

The purpose of this exercise is to see how your hand "sees" your face and how your face "feels" your hand. The connection will undoubtedly be stronger the next time you try this exercise. There is no need to judge the drawing, but you will definitely see improvement the next time around, when your hand and eye both learn to relax and coordinate their efforts in a tighter integration.

Fear

People who have frequent accidents often use these accidents as a "reason" for perpetuating their fear. It is as though *the accident justifies the fear*, and the two continually create each other.

The goal of this book is to help you become more aware and relaxed, to effectively organize movement and thought to improve physical performance and psychological bodies as instruments with which to make music. The human organism is delighted when given the opportunity to increase its playtime. We are in fact playing for time: the more often we play the more time we have for play—for activity, positive "growth" time. Imagine that the body is not only a wonderful musical instrument, but that there is a composer who plays through you.

Simplicity is the key. When you follow simple movments, it becomes easier to follow more complex movements. Mistakes are positive: they are to be learned from, and if you are concerned with "embarrassment" you can take heart from this simple truth. When embarrassment is dispensed with and mistakes seen as positive learning tools, the mental block is dissolved and the body follows along.

The Klutz is someone who blocks himself out of fear of failure, and who continually prepares himself for future failure with his thoughts. The Klutz has short-circuited the learning process, usually from some fear or other, substituting something totally inadequate.

Affirmation
I am safe in the world. Nothing is out to "get" me.

Exercise
If there is something relatively safe that you are afraid to do, try to overcome your irrational fears . . . by doing it.

Slipping

Slipping—as distinct from falling—usually occurs in the bathroom, which is perfectly natural since there is often water lying on the floor to "cause" an accident. Falling, on the other hand, can happen anywhere. Over the years, you may have come to see that it's not only water on the floor or in the tub that is responsible for bathroom accidents. The bathroom itself may conjure a certain predisposition, an attitude, if you will, that often recreates long suppressed memories and associations. Some of these associations may cause you to "go unconscious" in the bathroom and hurt yourself.

Affirmation

"I rejoice in all my memories, even the bad ones, since they are all vehicles for my learning experience." And: "I take care of myself in everything I do." (Best done completely relaxed in a nice hot bath.)

Exercises

1. Breathe in a connected, rhythmic pattern, in a hot bathtub, every night for a week. Let whatever memories come up, and then let them go with the next breath.

2. After your next bath or shower, rub off the excess water with your hands—before using the towel. Take your time, touch yourself gently or hard, feeling the consciousness of the body itself. Give yourself whatever feelings of love you think you either had or missed as a baby when you pat yourself dry with your towel.

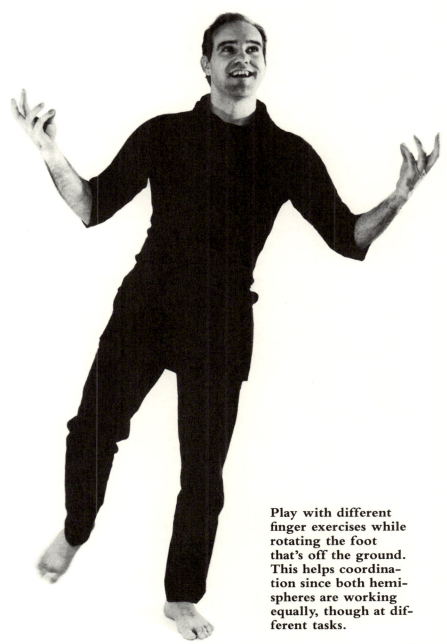

Play with different finger exercises while rotating the foot that's off the ground. This helps coordination since both hemispheres are working equally, though at different tasks.

Falling

Falling is a problem that gets more dangerous as you get older. Bones harden, muscles lose their elasticity, joints become arthritic, coordination lessens and you run the danger of injury from what would otherwise be considered normal activities. Numerous books on diet and fasting tell how to stop or even reverse the negative consequences of bad diet and poor exercise. We recommend a vegetarian diet that emphasizes raw food, raw vegetable juices, fruit, whole grains, sea vegetables, and occasionally fish. We also recommend the kinds of exercise that promote a healthy cardio-vascular system—walking, yoga, swimming, rope jumping—anything that is both enjoyable and gives the body a good workout. Hydrotherapy and sauna both promote cleansing and stimulate the heart and the eliminative organs.

However, for the prevention of falling, there are specific exercises that can be done daily which will improve your sense of balance. They should be done *together* with what has been mentioned before, and over time should reawaken the whole body to a new awareness of space and possibility.

Exercises

1. Alternate tip-toes. A good five-minute warm-up for feet and calves.

2. Walk in circles looking up. This promotes balance, brings up memories of early childhood.

3. Stand on one foot, holding the other.

4. "Tight-rope" walk on anything safe, like curbs, imaginary rope, etc.

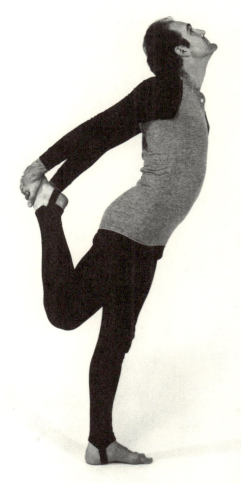

Hold one foot behind you, and arch your back as you look up.

Hemispheric Dominance

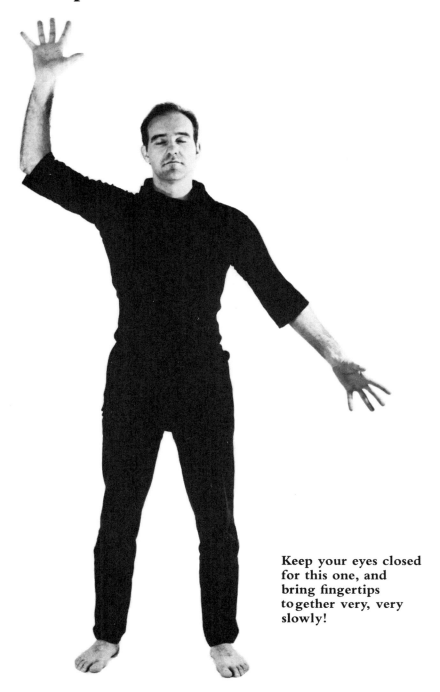

Keep your eyes closed for this one, and bring fingertips together very, very slowly!

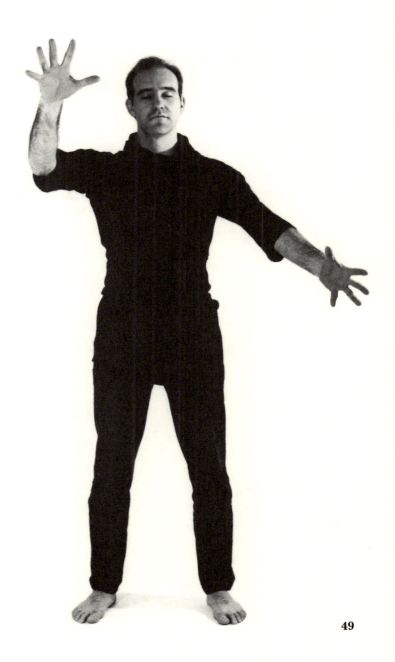

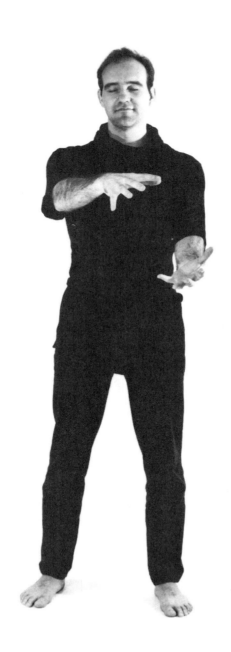

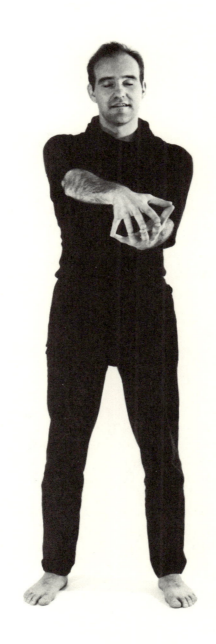

Most of us are not ambidextrous, and over time we use our less dominant hand less and less. Right-handed people use their right hands, left-handed people their left to the progressive exclusion of the other. Without use muscles will atrophy and the less dominant hand tends to lose whatever dexterity it had to begin with.

Moreover, studies show that ambidextrous people have more information passing between the two hemispheres of their brain, promoting greater overall functional integration. While not everyone can be ambidextrous, everyone can improve his/her ambidexterity, and gain physical agility in the process.

Affirmation
"Both sides of my body are working in perfect harmony."

Exercises
1. Strengthen your weaker eye by wearing an eye patch over the stronger eye every day for a few hours. Gradually the weaker eye will improve, and quite noticeably in some instances.

2. Write, draw, sign your name 100 times—with your "other" hand.

3. Squeeze a tennis ball with your "other" hand.

4. Wear a mitten or Ace bandage on your "good" hand, and let your "other" hand do *all the work* for a day or so, in a weekend.

Head Bumping

Pain is one way we have for waking up, and bumping your head can wake you up very quickly, indeed. The assumption is that most of us spend most of our waking moments not completely awake. Your clumsy part is that part which is literally in a "dream world." Living half awake is not all that bad; it is in large part a survival technique, keeping alive the part of us that is soft, relaxed, intuitive, right-brained. However, realize that when you *do* want to awaken and be more "in the moment" *you do not need pain to achieve it.* You can do it with pleasure as well—depending on your *attitude* not only towards your body but towards the "outside" world as well.

Affirmation
I enjoy giving and receiving pleasure during my waking hours.

Exercises

1. Lie on the floor, on your back, preferably on a soft carpet, and relax into your breathing. Massage your forehead with your left hand, and the back of your head with your right. Carry on for three or four minutes. Massage your eyes, brows, jaw, nose, mouth, temples, forehead, etc. Squeeze cheeks, eyebrows, chin. Reverse hands and continue.

2. Relax your head completely in the cups of your hands, and gently pass it back and forth between your hands, like the ball that it is. Play with the weight of it, letting the weight transfer freely. Feel the movement of the flesh and hair around the hardness of the skull.

3. Taking handfuls of hair very close to the scalp, pull gently for a few seconds. This will energize and vitalize the whole scalp, including nerve endings, stimulating circulation. Don't forget to maintain a slow rhythmic breathing pattern, relaxing on the exhale, pulling clear, strong, life-giving inhales.

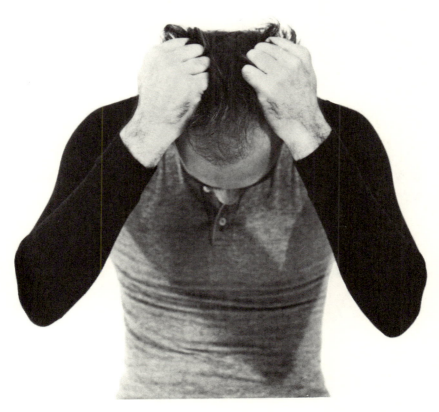

Fire

We all know that fire is hot, earth is solid, air is gaseous, and water is often wet. But we seldom allow ourselves to *experience* them. Therefore we may misread their cues and come into dangerous conflict with them. We have yet to learn as a civilization that nature is not to be conquered but to learn from and enjoy. And as individuals we have yet to learn that we have been given a body to learn *with* and enjoy, that consciousness is a state to be sought after rather than avoided.

Fire burns. You know that. Yet, why would you try to pick up a hot skillet with bare hands, even though there is a potholder, probably a cute one with embroidery, sitting on a nearby hook?

Quite possibly it has something to do with a mental block, established in childhood through fear and punishment. HOT! DON'T TOUCH! screamed the authority figure. So you retreat from experiencing fire, from learning its and your limits. You stop relating to hot things, stop, except in rare cases, working with them. You might sometimes develop defiant attitudes towards them, a kind of macho approach you sometimes find with welders. "I get burned all the time. It's no big thing"—kind of consciousness. Sometimes it has to do with an early curiosity that was never satisfied as to the nature of fire and heat. When you become "out of touch" with the elements is when they clamor for your attention—one way or another. It's as if they say to you: either experience us for the pleasure we give or experience the pain. You really have no choice other than to be conscious. The Prometheus myth is relevant here: Fire was/is sacred. It is a gift of the highest order.

Affirmation

I experience myself through the four elements. The more I experience the more I want to experience more.

Exercises

1. Meditate on a candle in your room every night for ten minutes. Let your thoughts go where they will, without becoming attached to any one thought. Notice them, and let them go. Appreciate the light from this one little candle. Feel the heat with your fingertip, the back of the hand, the palm of the hand. Experiment with the heat: feel it warm up your hand (from a safe distance). Recall your childhood fascination with fire. Recall the feeling that primitive people must have had towards the sacredness of fire. Think about how everything on this planet loves to combine with oxygen. Carbon loves oxygen. Why?

2. Burned tongues are no longer necessary. Whatever time you are taking to eat an average meal, double it, taking the extra time to taste everything and enjoy it. Hot drinks should be drunk from cups without handles. Follow the Chinese proverb: "too hot for hands, too hot for tongue."

3. Join a volunteer fire department and help rescue people and homes. Experience others' carelessness firsthand while sharpening your own powers of caring.

The Breath

The importance of the breath and breath control cannot be stressed strongly enough as a means for overcoming clumsiness. Connected, free breathing—breathing that releases held-on trauma and anxiety—can relax you to the point at which effective auto-suggestion is possible. Know what you want, and also know that it is possible to achieve. Various breathing techniques are effective in assisting the process of self-transformation. *Prana* yoga and Rebirthing are two that we know of, and there are teachers of these disciples in most cities in the United States.

Breathing is the most important thing you do every day, and every minute of the day. When you hold on to your breath, taking shallow inhales, holding on to anxiety in the process, you deny your body not only life-giving oxygen. More, you deny it *prana* or the electro-magnetic energy associated with every molecule in the Universe. When you hold your breath—*hypo*ventilate—you are holding on to a traumatic past, re-creating it in the present moment once again, somewhere in your body and mind. Freeing the breath helps you to free yourself from held-on tensions and anxieties, releasing mind and body to create the next moment as optimally as possible.

Affirmation
I am now breathing fully and freely.

Exercise
Notice your breath. When you have an anxious thought, notice how you hold your breath or breathe very shallowly. Whenever you find yourself holding your breath, notice the thought, take a deep inhale, relax the exhale and let go of the thought.

Breathing

T'ai Chi breathing is simple. The essence of the technique that the Taoists use is this: Inhale as you rise in movement, and exhale as you sink in movement. The inhalation comes in easily and naturally as you draw in your arms, and exhalation goes out as you extend your arms. Pushing movements are exhaled and pulling movements are inhaled.

Bending actions are accompanied by breathing out, and straightening actions are accompanied by breathing in. In this way you are connecting your movement to your breath and your breath to your movement, and likewise your thought processes will be connected to your breathing.

Thought and movement are one. As Hamlet says to the actors, "Suit the action to the word and the word to the action." A wonderful thing happens when we get an idea: we inhale and we say, "Aaahh!" Whenever we get an idea, we take in breath. Breathing is thinking, thinking is breathing. When we increase our breathing, we can increase our clarity of thinking. When we say "aaahh" we are in the expressive mode. We receive thoughts as we receive breath, and we express thoughts as we express breath.

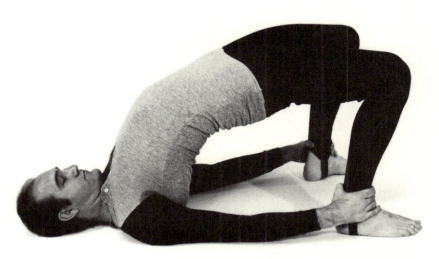

Notice the base of the throat, the location of the thyroid. Stay with your breath. Notice when you stop breathing, and start again.

Paralysis

We were walking down the street one night, observing the sights of an autumn in New York City, when we noticed a man in his 50's start to cross the street against the light. He had reached about a quarter of the way across when he noticed a car bearing down on him. He neither retreated to the curb, nor did he scurry across to the opposite side. He merely . . . stood there, paralyzed like a deer in the headlights of the oncoming car. We stopped and stared, fascinated by this display of infantile paralysis, and we don't mean polio. How fortunate we felt to be able to witness this scene, just as we were beginning to write this book, because it is a classic example, and, well, we were there. The man, for his part, was fortunate in that the car slowed down, stopped actually, and he released himself from his "frieze."

A major component of clumsiness is, of course, a kind of paralysis, a "holding on" that, carried to its extreme results in a complete cessation of motor control. In this state you literally cannot move when confronted with a major challenge, such as a car bearing down on you. Perhaps at some time in your life you were paralyzed, probably in fear. It entered your psyche and whatever it was that terrorized you initially, that terror has been kept somewhere handy where you can call on it when it is important that you do just the opposite.

Affirmation

I am safe in the world, and am creating safety for myself and others wherever I go.

Releasing Anger

If you feel you are a Klutz, realize that you are, in a way, the storm in the eye of calmness. If you are unable to express pain and anger, this leads to substituting clumsiness which leads to more pain and anger—like hitting your head, stubbing your toe or having an "accident." It is these actions that give you permission to actually express the pain that you were already feeling inside—*before the event*. Wouldn't it be easier, and safer to release those feelings before anyone gets hurt? Or do you want to carry pain and anger around with you?

Presuming that you don't, there are doorways through which you can release negative emotions without harming yourself or others.

Exercises

1. Rebirthing. This is a breathing technique during which negativity is released by connecting the inhale with the exhale until the breath begins breathing *you*. Never try this alone. There are hundreds of trained rebirthers all over the world who can guide you. If you do find yourself in a situation where you are hyperventilating spontaneously, keep breathing until you relax.

2. Create chaos in a safe space. Kick, scream and throw your arms and legs around in a temper tantrum. Call out to your "mother" to change your diapers. Kick and pound a bed with your hands and feet. If noise is a problem, scream into a pillow as loud as you can. This exercise will exhaust and relax you, bring you back into infantile repressions and rage and put you in touch with thoughts you might have had for decades.

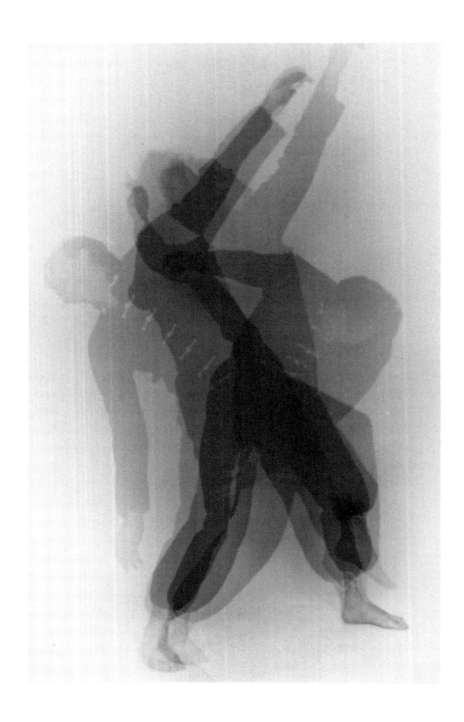

Chaos

When you exhibit Klutz behavior you are really looking for love and contact from others and the outside world. You walk into a room full of people and slip on a wet spot and are unable to organize a response quickly enough to avoid either falling or pulling a plate of canapes off the table nearby. As you do the dance of chaos you fly into the midst of laughter (a type of reward for clumsiness) *that is on one hand terribly upsetting and embarrassing and on the other hand a reward of attention by peers.* If the incident does not cause undue pain to the participant, the party jollies in the event and tension is released through laughter. If on the other hand the Klutz or someone else is injured enough to be a real problem you get a very different kind of attention. One is being laughed at and the other is being sympathized with. Either way, you as a Klutz have gotten attention, albeit negative. The problem is the fear of chaos and unintentionality so that as a Klutz you get little positive experience in allowing chaos to become positive.

An exercise that helps a Klutz to organize body/mind more efficiently is called "going into chaos." You need lots of space for this one, so make sure there is plenty of room for you to move about. For this is an exercise that it is helpful to have someone with you because you are going to give up control of your body and let it move through space in a totally random way. It is like falling but catching yourself at the last possible minute and then falling in a new direction. You can let out sound as you move. This can be in the form of words or in the form of shouts or screams or grunts and groans. This is a lot like being completely drunk and letting yourself fly about the space without regard to where you are going.

Let your arms fly in every direction and let your back and your legs go in any direction they want. The more chaotic you can allow yourself to be and *out of control you can feel*, the more control you will later be able to experience when you come back to your normal movements. The falling movements will allow you to feel that even in chaos there is a center that you can get in touch with and that you do have control enough to avoid actually falling all the way. The key to this exercise is to give in to the loss of control, to invest in loss as a strategy toward later gaining greater control of the body. Do this exercise for as long as you can keep it up. This is a physically demanding activity and you will feel washed out for a time. After you finish it the best thing is to sit still sixty seconds and then go into the exercise again for as long as you can take it. When you have allowed yourself the experience for a second time, sit for two minutes and catch your breath. As you sit, conscious of your breathing, focus your attention on ways in which you can let yourself go even more into an out-of-control state, letting all the juices flow like a great storm that comes in gusts and waves and has power and sound and fury. As you contemplate this last round of vigorous activity, note your breathing and what your feelings are telling you about your body. Go once more into the exercise if you can, and then rest. If you give yourself all you've got something strange and wonderful is likely to happen. You will experience long suppressed memories that will conjure up feelings of fear, rage, power, sexuality. Then you will feel once again in control. Chaos is a frightening state to most of us and that is why it is such a rich exercise to practice because the rewards are so high. In fact, the natural "high" you will get from this exercise will make you feel wonderful.

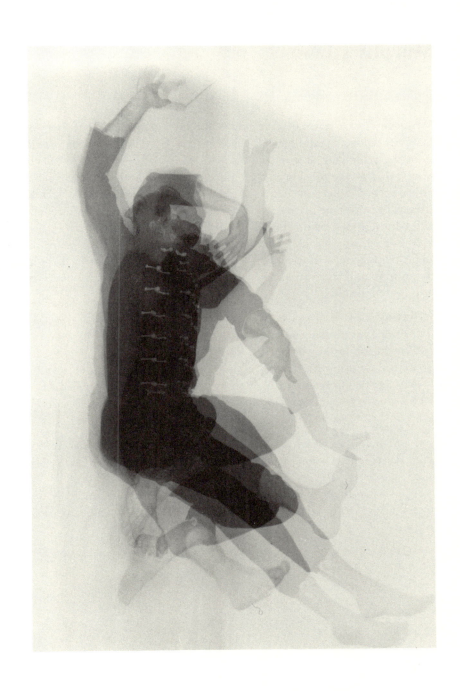

Murphy's Law

Murphy's Law states that anywhere you hurt yourself, at that spot you will hurt yourself again. Murphy, of course, was a Klutz. One reason that someone slaps you on your sunburn or that you stub your toe two or three times (same toe) or you get punched right where you have a bad bruise or cut is because your suffering is *attractive*, as in *magnetic*. Like attracts like. You are giving a signal that you want your pain noticed, and will continue that pain, or augment it until it is noticed.

Another reason has to do with repressed anger. Getting rid of repressed anger helps reduce the frequency of injury. Anger has a lot to do with frustration, and frustration not dealt with often becomes amplified until pain/injury result.

Affirmations

"I no longer need pain or injury to attract loving attention."
"Frustration no longer bothers me."
"I am now using my frustration to cure myself."
"My injury/clumsiness is a warning to take this book seriously."
"I love my body totally and my body loves me."

Exercises

1. Self-massage. Reach all over, especially neck, forearms and head.

2. Peripheral awareness eye exercises. Roll eyes slowly in ever-widening circles. Reverse direction.

3. Push-hands. With a partner, stand face to face. Place hands on each other's hands, palm to palm, and slowly move wherever the *hands* want to go.

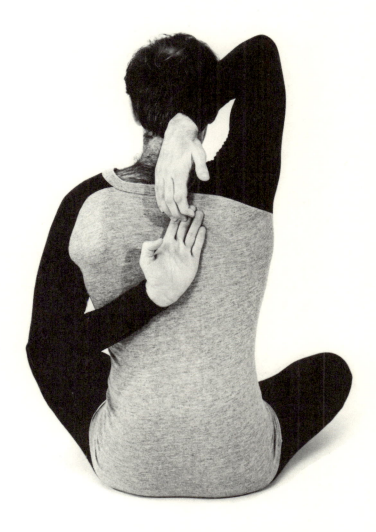

Grasp the fingers as shown and relax into the stretch. This exercise opens the chest and promotes feelings of safety. Stretch on alternate sides so that both get a good workout. If you can't link your hands behind your back, go as far as possible, gradually and gently.

Circulatory Stagnancy

Office workers, especially, are prone to accidents that arise from sitting all day and losing muscular and circulatory tone and elasticity. The following are offered in an effort to help correct this problem.

Exercises

1. Isometrics. Place both hands under desk while seated. Press up against the bottom of the desk for a count of ten. Gradually increase the amount of pressure you're exerting as well as the time allotted.

2. Still seated, place hands between your knees and try to force the knees inwards against your hands, while exerting a counter pressure against your knees with the hands. Follow as before.

3. Now, reverse the hands and knees, placing hands on the outside of your knees and try to force your legs together, while exerting an outward pressure against the hands.

4. Invent your own exercise. The main obstacle towards better health and a livelier circulation is entropy. Entropy is doing something—or not doing something—because that's the way it's always been done. Overcoming physical stagnancy begins with overcoming mental stagnancy.

Office exercises can be done without sacrificing work-time. In fact, they offer the prospect of greater efficiency from the onset.

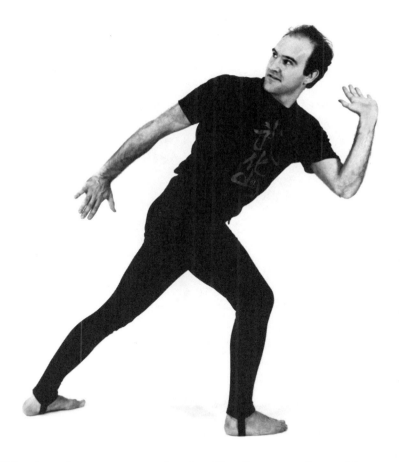

This gives the torso a good twist. Slowly rotate from side to side.

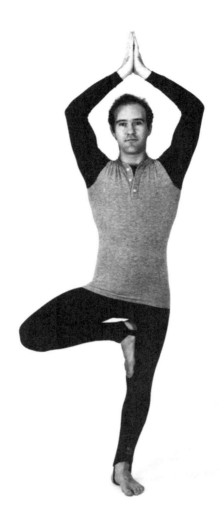

Standing on one foot, set the heel of your other foot on the inside of your thigh. Place palms together and raise them above your head. Repeat with opposite legs.

Circulatory Stagnancy II

People in offices tend to lead sedentary lives, and this has given rise to tremendous health problems, including "bad backs," poor circulation, loss of muscle tone, premature aging and, of course, "clumsiness." If you are in this kind of situation, and are a normally agile person, over time you will lose your agility from living/coping with an unnatural environment. All day sitting in indoor light, stale air, synthetic surroundings—despite the decorative plants—tobacco and coffee, add up to a prescription for accidents.

Here are some five-minute stretches that will invigorate and empower the system, energize it and restore lost vitality. They will prevent fatigue due to stagnation and will help you oxygenate your bloodstream.

Exercises

1. Neckroll. To prevent stiffness in your neck and upper back, roll your head in slow circles, three times one way, then three times the other way. Feel the pull in shoulders. This can be accompanied by a neck twist in which you turn your head and look over your shoulder, keeping your body facing forward.

2. Spinal twist in chair. With your feet planted firmly on the floor, slowly bring the upper body around, grasping the back of the chair if possible until the top part of you is turned as far as it will go in one direction. Hold it for a minute or so and then slowly come back to a normal sitting position. Then reverse direction.

3. In a standing position, lean back, hands on hips. Lean back as far as you can comfortably and hold it. This should work the stomach muscles. You can rotate the hips to vary this one.

4. Knee to chest. While in a sitting position, you can give the lower back a good stretch by simply bringing the knees to the chest one at a time. Grasp each knee with both hands, interlocking the fingers.

5. Tension shake-out. Let the arms dangle while in a standing position. Slowly start to shake out the hands, with wrists and forearms completely relaxed. Some tension should drain from the fingers, thereby improving your typing and outlook. Gradually increase the speed of shaking.

Losing

Everyone has a friend who is forever losing things, usually keys, address books, sometimes wallets, whatever. They are at "sixes and sevens." They bump into things looking for whatever it is they lost. They would be funny if their cases weren't so pathetic. They are scattered and . . . they make their things *disappear*. Perhaps you are such a person; most people have their . . . phases.

The point is that there seems to be a correlation between losing important things like keys and address books, and your physical adroitness, dexterity. Such people are "all thumbs." They scatter themselves and their possessions wherever they go. It's as though they create a whirlwind, and they and their things fly off the periphery. The *I Ching* often counsels to keep still in such situations when it does not further to cross "great waters."

Affirmations

My mind is still as a deep lake. I have continuous access to whatever it is I need.

Exercises

1. Create a whirlwind with your body, flailing arms. Spin, thrash and/or kick. Mess your hair, using your hands as eggbeaters. Stick out your tongue, roll it around your mouth and make sounds instead of words.

2. Stop. Sit very still. Turn off the lights. Feel the whirlwind dissipate and calm return gradually. Relax on the exhales with your eyes gently closed. As you feel the calm, register the feeling. It's yours to keep wherever you are.

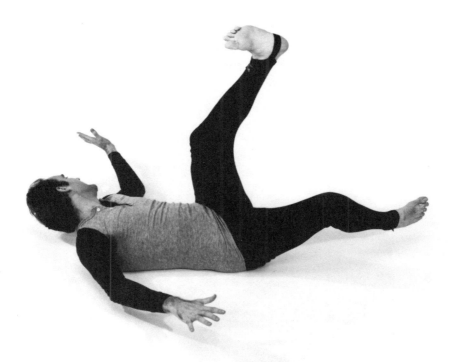

Roll around and flail. When you stop, you'll feel relaxed enough to start organizing.

Guilt

Many a Klutz there is who is trying to punish him/herself for a 30-year-old "sin." If that sin went unpunished, the Klutz then takes on the role of avenging authority to punish himself—usually on a continuous basis. If the original transgression was punished, the adult Klutz will also keep on punishing himself, especially if the original "sin" was to be born in the first place, or being born the "wrong" sex, if the parents wanted something else. The only exit from this predicament is total forgiveness.

Affirmations

"I forgive my parents totally for being ignorant and cruel."

"I forgive myself totally for hurting myself."

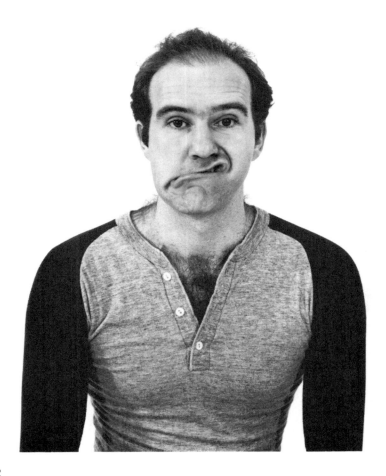

Embarrassment

The person beset by clumsiness is often a person in perpetual embarrassment. A lifetime of derision, concealed laughter and condescension by gym teachers often produces an ugly duckling who cannot make the leap to beautiful swan. A shell begins to grow at an early age, and it calcifies over time into a person grown accustomed to attenuated existence.

Affirmations
"I no longer need or seek the approval of others since the Universe itself gives me everything I need."

"My mind and body are in continuous harmony with themselves and with every aspect of physical existence."

Exercises
1. Make faces in the mirror. 5 minutes a day.
2. Volunteer to work with the handicapped.
3. Sing a song for someone or recite a poem on the street. The next time you feel embarrassed to do something, do it. If someone else you're with embarrasses you, remember to tell yourself and others what the truth is as you see it if that's feasible; also judgeth not that ye be not judged.

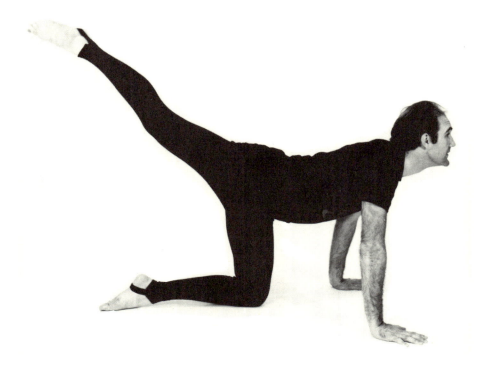

On your hands and knees, bring your knee and head together and then arch your head upwards as you extend your leg into the air. Repeat to both sides. This strengthens the back and helps timing and coordination.

Timing

The Klutz always tries to do the "right thing." It is better to align yourself with whatever is happening. The key word here is "trying." What the Klutz is doing is trying. Many people try to, say, quit smoking. They do not quit. They *try* to quit, and therefore never actually quit. There is an analogy here with the Klutz who is continually trying to get it—whatever "it" happens to be—*right*. Implicated in all this is an effort to please someone else, a parent or a teacher perhaps.

There is a certain magic in the clumsy person's dream-like world, a magic that is often intrinsically endearing, and something that elicits genuine feelings of warmth from others more physcially coordinated. This magic enables certain things to happen for the Klutz, unintended positive consequences, as when things go right, in spite of everything.

But sometimes this leads you into a false sense of "security," believing that you can muddle through, regardless. And you go right on trying, because sometimes this trying works.

Affirmation
I deserve love.

Exercises
1. Pleasing yourself. A certain amount of time/money should be set aside for pleasuring yourself. A once a week massage, for example, or a health club membership.

2. A reachable goal—such as any one of the exercises in this book—should be accomplished and then noted as a success, logged in the record of things done, rather than things *tried*. Know, too, that the magic that enables a certain modicum of success in the world will not only continue, but will become enhanced by the effort undertaken to pleasure yourself.

3. All disapproving messages coming from parents/teachers from years ago should be noted, then put right by the above affimation.

Timing II

Part of being clumsy is the result of being shut off from your own natural rhythms. The Klutz will almost always be unable to keep anything more than a simple 4/4 rhythm and sometimes not even that. The body just doesn't "hear" it, and is unable to "follow" it.

Exercises

1. Alternate nostril breathing (*nadi-suti*). This calms the nerves and enables you to get in touch with some natural inner rhythms that go on all the time.

2. Play a game of Jacks. A good game of Jacks can be of immense help in establishing timing.

3. Juggle with one ball. Then two. Then three. But start with one and do it for a few minutes a day.

4. Listen to and tell some good jokes. Your sense of timing will develop through an appreciation for the funny part, which is more than half timing.

5. Trust a partner. (Fall into the arms of your partner, etc.) This is de-rigidifying.

6. Play video games, excellent for eye-hand coordination. A few pennies buys you timing.

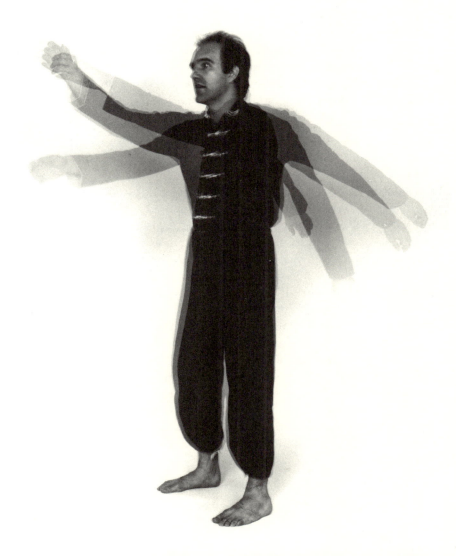

This relaxes the arms and gets the blood moving. A surprisingly simple, yet effective way to get the body going. Allow the torso to turn as it will.

Timing III

Awkwardness is the cumulative result of trying to live somewhere else than in the present. If this book is about anything it is about *inhabiting the moment*, and claiming it for life itself. Gracefulness is about being in the totality of life, and if life is not to be lived, what's the point?

So the problem here is still one of *timing*. Timing can be improved in hundreds of ways, all of them enjoyable and fulfilling.

Exercises

1. *Dance to your own drummer*. Grace and timing come when you live at peace with your own life force. Music and rhythm help this come about. Dance and sing whenever you have the thought to. Overcoming awkwardness is also overcoming inhibitions, shyness, "self-consciousness." It's okay to be conscious of yourself so long as this consciousness does not lead to self-suppression. Finger dancing is great, too, and foot tapping, and counting the rhythm inside. Claim some time alone if you have to, put on the record and twirl your hips and stamp those feet. Direct your appreciation to the music *within*. If you don't like what you're feeling, change the record!

2. With a partner, mirror each other's movements. Let one of you lead for ten minutes and then let the other person lead. The movements do not have to be stylized—they can be very natural. The important thing here is to get into each other's rhythms.

3. Continuing with the preceding exercise let yourselves introduce sounds and words. Talk as you play. The leader's responsibility is to be as easy to follow as possible, and to establish a contact, gain attention and a degree of concentration that is not easily broken. The follower's responsibility is to observe and follow as closely and precisely the movements and sounds of the leader, as is possible.

4. In the bathtub lie on your back with your knees bent and the water coming up to just under your chin. Begin breathing deeply, and watch the water as the level in the tub begins to take on the rhythm of your breathing. Once there is a wave pattern set up in the tub, try to maintain the rhythm of this wave. Try to attune your breathing to the movement of the wave and gradually increase the size of the wave, as if pushing a swing. As the wave gets more powerful and higher, your breathing will also become more powerful and deeper. Just as a swing goes higher and higher, and you have to stay in synch with its movements so do you have to keep yourself in synch with the wave that you started with your breath.

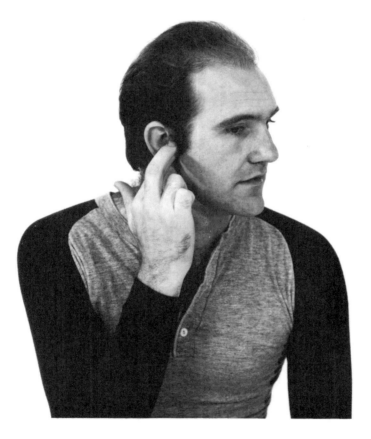

With your index finger, close the "little door" to your ear and tap with your middle finger. Don't ask why. It does work, though, to remind you to listen better.

Not Listening

It is an old adage that the body never lies. Accidents, both major and minor, are messages from the body that something is wrong and needs correction. Failing to listen to that message means that your body has to repeat itself until you listen. In this day of Damoclean precariousness, famine and impending plague, the obligation of the entire species is to wake up to the messages coming in. Since the dawning of the nuclear age there have been thousands of nuclear "accidents" that have gone unheeded by the body politic.

If we heed the lessons of the little accidents along the way we can avoid the bigger ones later. Again, it's a question of attitude. Why is it so hard for this species to learn from its mistakes? People seem to have a gigantic learning disability that keeps the entire civilization in a situation of repeating past mistakes over the centuries, trying to avoid the consequences of bad thinking. The world promotes bad ideas in the name of profit, national pride or winning, while the major priorities of survival, health, personal or cultural fulfillment are often neglected. This happens when meaning is distorted, allowing for the lies and denigration to continue. We say one thing and mean another. Then we wonder what the "meaning of life" is.

Habit

Accidents are often the result of habitual movement—movement that takes place while the body is functionally asleep. While much habitual movement is functional, some is dangerous. The body has a knowledge all its own, carrying on while the ego or the mind is working on other things. Patterned behavior helps carry you along and you quite appropriately rely on your body to take you where you want to go. However, when there is too much noise in your head, too many distractions or anxiety, when your body/mind is preoccupied, danger cannot be far behind.

Affirmation

"Injury and illness decrease in proportion to my love for and awareness of my body."

Exercises

1. Blindfold yourself and sit at a table. Arrange different objects, or play with those already there. Still blindfolded, walk around a very safe room. Bring your hands together from a variety of angles and try to make your fingertips touch at the first pass. Start slowly and gather speed. For example, bring your left hand down from the top of your head and try to meet your right hand which you bring up from behind your hip.

2. On a track, beach, etc., run backwards.

3. Breaking patterns helps the body keep from rusting. Notice your patterned movements and invent new ways for doing old chores.

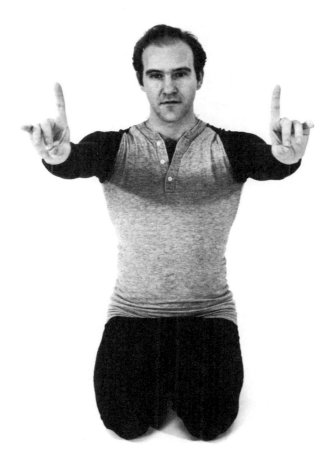

Closing one eye, hold out one hand with your finger pointing towards the ceiling. You will soon find a "blind spot" where part of the finger actually disappears.

Tension in the Arms

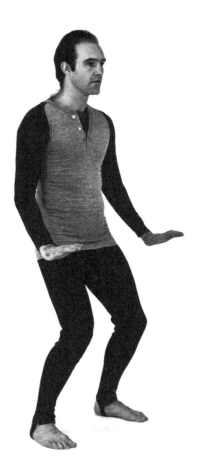

Very slowly, raise your arms from your thighs to above your head and back down to your thighs in a wave-like motion. Then, shake out your hands, until they're completely relaxed. Repeat.

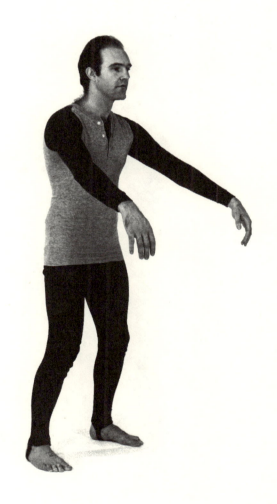

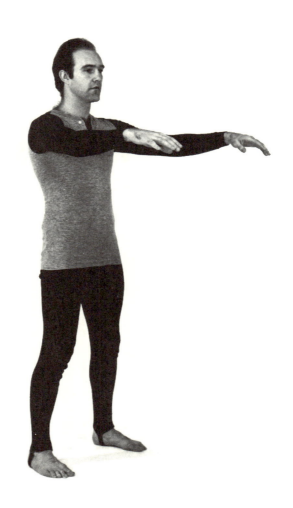

Manual dexterity is heavily influenced by the tension or lack of it in the arms, as well as shoulders and back. One sure-fire way of releasing held-on tension in the arms is to stand up with the eyes closed, and bounce up and down on your toes, shoulders and arms completely relaxed. Let your arms bounce up and down with the rest of the body, and let the head roll freely. With your wrists completely relaxed, shake your hands up and down and let the tension pour out of the fingers. Don't forget to breathe rhythmically and keep your knees slightly bent.

Make a fist, squeezing as hard as you can. Hold it as long as you can, then relax your hands. Tighten all the muscles in your arms, shoulders, back, pelvis, legs and feet, one muscle group at a time. Then relax. Do the same with your face, scrunching it up, holding it, and then relaxing. This exercise will relax your entire body, giving it energy at the same time. This is good for any time during the day.

Lateness

Grace and precision are the result of moving in harmony with the world as it is. Lateness is clumsiness in the social realm. It is often the result of an attitude that assumes that your time is more important than someone else's. In the highest sense giving and receiving are the same, since the giver ideally takes as much pleasure (from giving) as the receiver. Being habitually late is evidence of a taker, someone who has set up an *unequal* posture vis-à-vis the rest of the world, and since the world is a reciprocating place, the taker will find other people who want to take from him.

Affirmation

"My coordinating improves in my own body as I coordinate on an equal basis with other people."

Going Unconscious

Movement and consciousness go hand in hand. Space/time and body/mind have a certain equivalency. Movement in the mind precedes movement in the body. Or to put it another way, the body/mind is always moving. This book is about coordinating the body/mind, funneling consciousness to useful purpose.

Exercises

1. While jogging, count the rhythm of the breath. Make playful changes, such as alternating rhythms of 3:4 and 4:4, or 11:16, whatever. This develops the consciousness derived from getting in close touch with the breath.

2. While jogging, count your heartbeats and get in touch with your heart. This will actually exercise the part of your brain that is directly in synch with your heart. You get more tuned in.

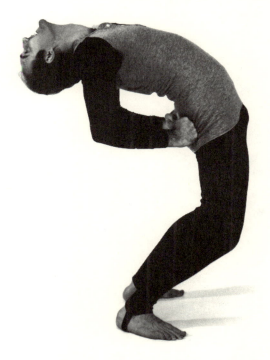

Bend back all the way, as shown. Hold it. Become conscious of everything in your body. Come up slowly and repeat.

Masks

Every one of us wears a mask to some degree or another. You probably have a work mask, a social mask, a party mask, an "I'm innocent" mask, or a tough guy mask. These masks are functioning throughout the day without your really taking the time to see how they keep you from being as graceful as you really can be. Because they are frozen and keep you trapped behind restricted movement and expressions. You respond habitually to external events. This increases the potential for danger, since masks help keep reality at a distance. In order to put you in touch with these masks and to make you more aware of when they are activated you can play with them.

1. In front of a mirror make as many different faces as you can. Then, as you watch the changes, hold one face that is familiar to you for as long as you can without changing it. Do this with as many of these faces/masks as you can for as long as your face muscles can hold out.

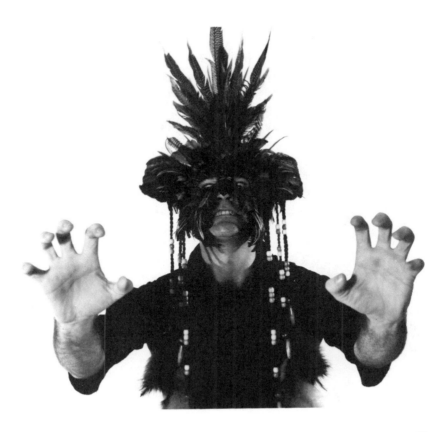

2. Get several different masks. They can be Halloween masks or the see-through variety, or any kind. Choose one and hold it in front of you. Stare at it for several minutes. Examine it. How does it make you feel? Is it sad? Is it happy? Really study it and let it come inside you. Put it on and close your eyes. Imagine that the mask is alive and that you are this person or creature. How does it breathe? What does it feel like to be this person? After a few minutes of going through these questions in your mind open your eyes and look in the mirror, which should be close by. Let your body take on the physicality of this other person of this mask. Let the deep psychological state of this person come out through you. It may be funny or it may be very serious. Let it be what it is. Let the mask have total freedom to act in any way it wants to. Don't be afraid. Let this person explore your house or room and touch things. Often a mask will be like a child—sometimes very friendly, sometimes very hostile. Allow this to come out. What a mask does is allow us to get in touch with those parts of ourselves that we may have shut down when we were children. Therefore they are part of us and need to be let out so that they don't get us in trouble by making us clumsy.

3. Jump up and down, with or without a jumprope.

4. Allow yourself to play an association game by saying any word that comes to mind and associate that word with another that leads you to another. Let the flow of words come tumbling out so that you can begin to let the words come out whenever they like. Let them surprise you. Surprise yourself with sounds too. You don't have to just use words.

5. Repeat the above exercise doing it with your body. Let one part move and let another respond and then let another movement arise out of that and let the movements take you anywhere they want to.

6. Jump up and clap. The best way to rid oneself of habitual thinking, especially the kind that identifies with suffering, is to choose new models.

7. Choose a mythological hero who through some difficulty reaches a desired new state. Close your eyes after getting to know the story and see yourself as this hero, or heroine, acting out the story. Next, get up in front of a mirror and act out all the movement as if it were a movie or a dance until you defeat the monster or you win the battle or achieve the goal.

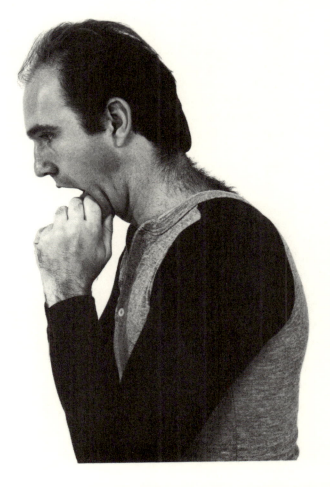

Relax your jaw and wiggle it with your hand. This helps relax the entire face and makes you aware of how you may be posing your mouth.

8. Choosing a painting from one of the great masters that exhibits to you the most graceful and the most elegant and the most relaxed position. Now imagine yourself as the model of who is pictured. Place yourself in this position and sit for the artist. Stay in this position for several minutes and then relax. Continue to keep the fantasy of gracefulness alive in your movements as you go from the posing to your natural position.

9. Choose an athlete you feel is extraordinarily graceful. Watch this athlete on television and then imitate some of his/her movements. All of these exercises will help give you a new vision of yourself and can aid you in changing your self image. They will give you conscious models on which you can draw to give you a new perspective on your body and its use.

"To thine own self be true and it must follow as the night the day thou canst not then be false to any man," says Polonius to Laertes in *Hamlet*. Being false can lead you to many "unlucky" incidents. It makes you uncomfortable with the people you lie to and also on some level makes you the source of discomfort to those to whom you have given false impressions. The body never lies. Telling the truth to yourself helps you to bring ability and the ease of grace to the body and the ease and simplicity of concentration to greater heights. The truth does set you free.

Exercises

1. Standing in front of a mirror, recount to yourself some important lies you have told. Tell yourself what it was you were hiding and what you gained by lying. Now proceed to tell a lie to yourself and see what you feel about watching yourself as you lie to yourself. Next, tell the truth about the same subject, and see how that feels. Which feels better?

2. In front of a mirror go through all the lies you can remember and pretend that you are with the people to whom you lied and tell them the truth and ask them for forgiveness for having lied. Visualize their forgiving you.

About the Authors

David Chandler is an actor, choreographer, and martial artist. He has worked extensively in New York City theatre and has staged fight scenes both in the United States and in the Netherlands. He has taught T'ai Chi for the past eight years, in part under a Ford Foundation grant at the INTAR Theatre. He is currently teaching movement for actors at the Ensemble Studio Theatre Institute. He has led workshops in movement, T'ai Chi and stage combat extensively in this country and abroad. In 1985, he was the staff T'ai Chi instructor at the Omega Institute for Holistic Studies. Mr. Chandler leads workshops for businesses to increase productivity and reduce accidents in the workplace. He overcame his own personal Klutz through athletics and the use of these exercises.

Jonathan Eisen, Editorial Director of Sterling IMPACT Books, is the author of several books, including *Unknown California* (Macmillan) and *The Nobel Reader* (Clarkson N. Potter). He is a student of Hatha Yoga and Rebirthing.

J. B. Grant has been a catalogue photographer for L. L. Bean, Montgomery Ward, J. C. Penney, and others. As a nature photographer he won First Place Award for Excellence in Photography by the Sierra Club. He also does interior design and architectural photography. This is his first book.

Index

Accident(s), 11
  habitual, 82
  -prone, 11
Air, 54
Ambidextrous, 52
Anger, 59
Arthritis, 46
Attitude, 12
Awareness, 9
  kinesthetic, 34

Balance, 27, 29, 30, 33
Believing, 11
Blockage, 35
Breath, 56, 57, 59, 76

Canoes, 8
Cardio-vascular system, 46
Chaos, 61
Childhood, re-experiencing 30, 39
Circulatory system, 66, 69
Clumsiness, as blockage, 35
Communication, 33
Consciousness, 88
Control, conscious, 32
Coordination, 88

Dance, 78
Dominance, hemispheric, 48
Drawing, 42

Earth, 24, 54
Elderly, 14
Embarrassment, 18, 73
Evaluation, self-, 16

Falling, 46
Fear, 43
Fingers, 40
Fire, 54
Forgiveness, 26, 72
Free, 27
Frustration, 18

Grace, 78
Groundness, 24

Hamlet, 94
Headstrong, 18

I Ching, 70
Imbalance, physical, 27
Inhibition, 39
Injury, head, 52
Introspection, 34

Joy, 27

Labels, personal, 36
Lateness, 88
Losing, 70
Love, 38

Magic, 75
Masks, social, 90
Massage, 29, 40, 64
Mistakes, as learning tools, 43
Murphy's Law, 64
Muscle elasticity, 46
Music, 78

Overcompensating, 32
Oxygen, 56, 69

Pain, 59, 64
Paralysis, 58
Pleasure, 75
Power, personal, 15, 16, 37, 62
Prana, 56
Proving, need for, 19, 20

Rebirthing, 59

Security, 75
Sin, original, 72
Slipping, 44
Spine, 22
Spinning, 30
Spontaneity, 39
Suffering, 92

T'ai Chi, 57
Tension, 13, 22, 69, 87
  in the arms, 84
Timing, 75, 76, 78

Water, 54